The Vibrant Dash Diet Cooking Plan

50+ Tasty Recipes for Everybody

Zoe Kimmel

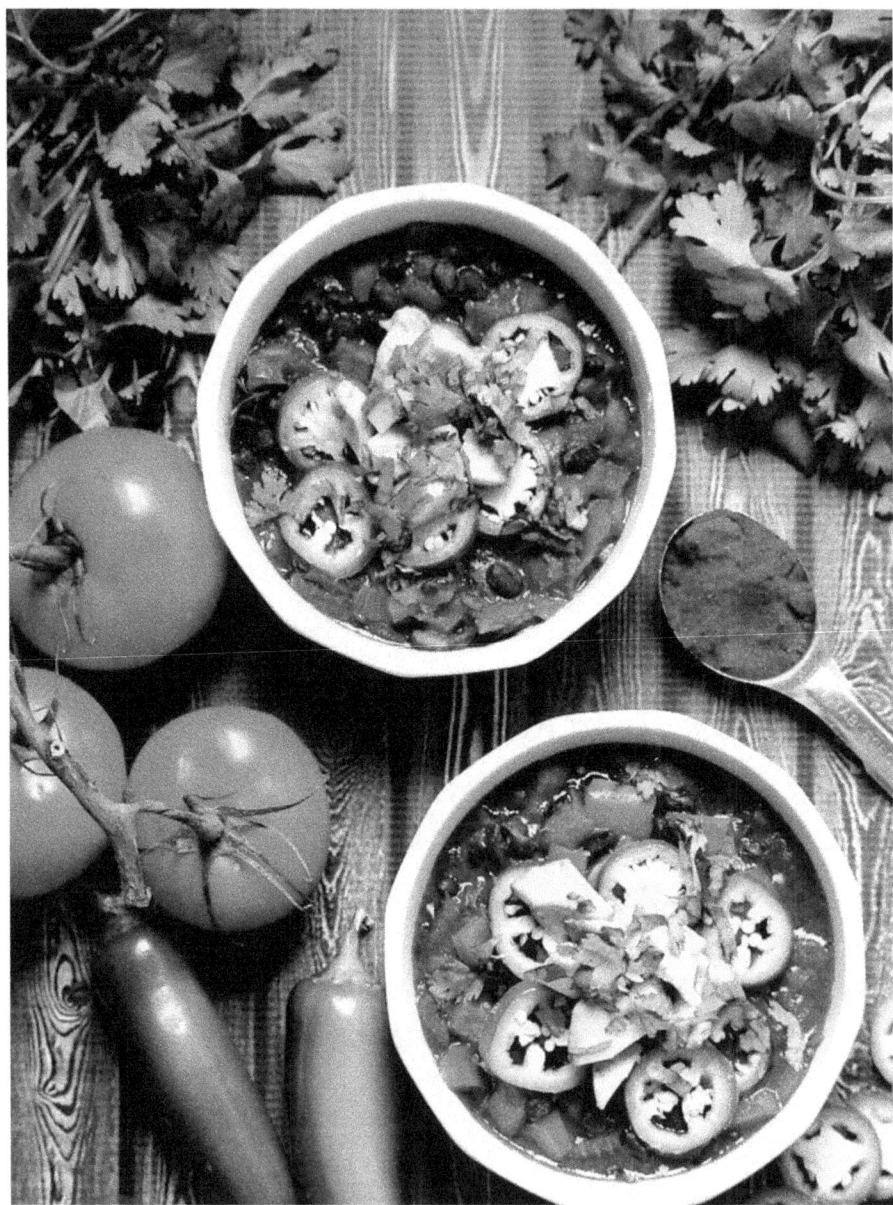

Table of Contents

Sugar Break Apple and Peanut Butter Oatmeal

Ingredients

1 cup steel-cut oats

Three medium-large Granny Smith apples, cored and sliced into 1-2" chunks

A swirl of peanut butter

pinch ground cinnamon

1 tbsp butter (optional)

4 cups of water

pinch salt

Directions

Cook the oats till they reach the specified texture and creaminess.

Cut apples, toss them into the oats, and stir.

Then add spread into it and stir until melted and spread throughout.

Top with a touch of cinnamon and butter (optional) and enjoy!

Nutrient Calories: 453

Sweet Potato Toast

Ingredients

One potato (sweet)

Instructions

1.   Divide the sweet potato into 1/4-inch slices and pop into the toaster.

2.   Top with anything you select. Popular combinations include spread with fruit, avocado, hummus, eggs, cheese, and tuna fish salad.

Nutrient Calories: 112

Ulli's Granelli

Ingredients

4 cups rolled oats

2 cups raw cashews

2 cups raw walnuts

2 cups of raw almonds

2 cups of fresh sunflower seed

2 cups of raw pumpkin seeds

3 cups unsweetened coconut flakes

1/2 cup of maple liquid syrup

1/4 cup of unrefined coconut oil, plus 2 tsp for oiling the baking sheet

pinch of sea salt

1/3 cup of pure orange oil

2 cups of organic raisins

2 cups of dried cherries or cranberries

Directions

1.   Set the oven to 300°F.

2.   during a considerable bowl, mix the oats, nuts, seeds, and coconut flakes.

3.   Take a little bowl, stir together the syrup, copra oil, salt, and orange oil till well combined, then pour over the oat-nut combination and blend nicely.

4.   Spread granola on an outsized oiled baking sheet (do it in batches if needed) and bake for 35-forty minutes until golden brown (rotate the baking sheet halfway via for even baking).

5.   Remove from oven and permit refreshing absolutely before mixing with raisins and dried cherries or cranberries.

6.   Store in airtight place within the fridge to stay extra crispiness.

Tofu Turmeric Scramble

Ingredients

One 8-ounce block of firm or extra-firm tofu, drained 1 tbsp extra virgin olive oil ¼ red onion, chopped

One green or purple bell pepper, chopped 2 cups of clean spinach, loosely chopped ½ cup sliced button mushrooms ½ tsp every salt and pepper

1 tsp garlic powder

½ tbsp turmeric

¼ cup nutritional yeast

Directions

1.   Drain the tofu and squeeze lightly to try to to away with extra water. Crumble tofu right into a bowl with the help of hand - the smaller the pieces, the higher.

2.   Prep vegetables and region an outsized skillet at medium temperature. Once ready, then add vegetable oil, onions, and bell peppers. Mix during a pinch of the salt and pepper and prepare dinner for about five minutes to melt the vegetables. Then add mushrooms and sauté for two mins. Then upload tofu. Sauté for about three minutes, a touch more if the tofu is watery.

3.   Add the remainder of the salt, pepper, garlic turmeric, and nutritional yeast and blend with a spatula, ensuring the spices combo well. Cook for an additional 5 to eight mins till tofu is lightly browned.

4.   Add the spinach and canopy the pan so as to steam for 2 minutes. Serve immediately with facets of your choice.

Nutrient Calories: 158

Whole Grain Cheese Pancakes

Ingredients

1 cup of oat flour

1/2 cup of sorghum flour

2 tbsp of teff flour

1/3 cup of plus 1 tbsp, tapioca starch

1 tbsp of baking powder

1/2 of tsp salt

3 1/2 of tsp sugar

1/2 tsp of flax meal

3/4 cup of buttermilk

1/3 cup of cottage cheese

Three eggs

half tsp vanilla extract

4 tsp canola oil

1-pint blueberries

1/2 cup maple syrup

3 tbsp water

1 tsp lemon juice

pinch of salt

Instructions

1.   Combine all of your dry elements during a huge bowl and stir to combine evenly.

2.   Whisk all of your wet ingredients in another bowl collectively.

3.   Make a hole within the center of your dry substances and start to slowly pour within the wet materials, a few quarter cup at a time. this may confirm that no lumps form when whisking.

4.   Continue including your wet components to the flour base till a smooth batter form. Let the batter relax for quarter-hour at an equivalent time as you preheat your grill.

5.   While the grill is warming up, make a warm maple blueberry compote. Mix blueberries, syrup, water, lemon juice, and a pinch salt during a small pot. Stir frivolously to combine.

6.   Gently heat the pot over medium-low warmth till the blueberries start to pop and release their natural juices. Set aside, but maintain heat.

7.   Once the grill is preheated to a medium-hot temperature, lightly oil the restaurant employing a nonstick spray or a small amount of neutral-flavored oil.

8.   Ladle the batter on to the skillet, ensuring you are doing not overload it.

9.   Give time to the pancakes to cook undisturbed until the looks of the sides dry and bubbles come to the surface without breaking. This has got to take roughly minutes.

10.   Flip the pancakes over and cook at the opposite facet for an additional two minutes.

11.   Keep heat or serve immediately with the sweet and comfy maple-blueberry compote.

Nutrient Calories: 511

Red Pepper, Kale, and Cheddar Frittata

Ingredients

1 tsp olive oil

5 oz baby kale and spinach

One red pepper, diced

1/3 cup sliced scallions

12 eggs

3/4 cup milk

1 cup sharp shredded cheddar cheese

1/4 tsp salt

1/4 tsp pepper

Directions

1.   Preheat oven to 375 □.

2.   Spray an eight 1/2-inch by using 12-inch glass or casserole dish with vegetable oil or nonstick spray.

3.   Heat oil during a large frypan. Add crimson peppers on low and cook until tender. Add kale and spinach, on occasion stirring till vegetables are wilted, or for about three min.

4.   Transfer peppers and greens to the plate, spreading evenly. Add sliced scallions.

5.   Beat eggs with milk, salt, and pepper. Pour the egg aggregate over the pan. Sprinkle cheese on top.

6.   Bake about 35-40 mins or till the mixture is totally set and starting to lightly brown. For extra color, place under broiler for an extra 1 to 3 minutes, watching to make sure the highest doesn't burn. Let cool about five mins before cutting it.

7.   Serve it as warm or refrigerate for a fast breakfast during the week

— microwave for 1-2 minutes to reheat.

Nutrient Calories: 77

Scrambled Eggs with Bell Pepper and Feta

Ingredients

Olive oil-Salad or cooking-1 tsp-4.5 grams

Green bell pepper-Sweet, green, raw-2 medium (approx 2-3/4"

long, 2-1/2" dia)-238 grams Egg-Whole, fresh eggs-Four large-200 grams Feta cheese-1 oz-28.4 grams

Directions

1.   Heat the oil during a skillet on medium heat. Add chopped peppers and cook till tender.

2.   Stir the eggs and increase the skillet with the peppers. Stir slowly over medium-low heat till they attain your preferred doneness. Sprinkle inside the feta cheese and stir to combine and soften the cheese. Serve directly and luxuriate in it!

Nutrient

Calories 448 Carbs 14g Fat 30g Protein 31g Fiber 4g Net carbs 10g Sodium 551mg Cholesterol 769mg

Devilled Egg Toast

Ingredients

Egg-Whole, fresh eggs-Two large-100 grams Mustard-Prepared, yellow-2 tbsp-30 grams

Light mayonnaise-Salad dressing, Kraft brand-2 tbsp-30 grams Whole-wheat bread-Commercially prepared-Four slice-112 grams

Directions

1.   Place egg during a bowl and canopy with water. Boil the water, remove from heat, cover, and let sit 10 minutes. Drain under cold water, peel, and mash.

2.   Combine egg with the mustard and mayonnaise. Mix well.

3.   Toast bread and top with egg mixture. Enjoy!

Nutrition

Calories 543 Carbs 53g Fat 24g Protein 28g Fiber 8g Net carbs 45g Sodium 1173mg Cholesterol 382mg

Basic Scrambled Eggs

Ingredients

Egg-Whole, fresh eggs-Six large-300 grams

Butter-Unsalted-1 tbsp-14.2 grams

Chives-Raw-1 tbsp chopped-3 grams

Tarragon-Spices, dried-1 tbsp, ground-4.8 grams

Table-One dash-0.40 grams

Pepper-Spices, black-One dash-0.10 grams

Directions

1.   Beat the eggs during a bowl and till damaged up. Sprinkle with a pinch each of salt and pepper and beat to include. Place tablespoons of the eggs during a small bowl; put aside.

2.   Heat a 10-inch nonstick frypan over medium-low warmth until hot, approximately 2 minutes. Add butter to the pan and therefore the usage of a rubber spatula, swirl until it's melted and foamy, and therefore the box is flippantly coated. Pour within the massive a part of the eggs, sprinkle with chives and tarragon (if the usage of), and let sit down undisturbed till eggs just start to line round the edges, about 1 to 2 minutes. Using the rubber spatula, push the eggs from the edges into the center .

After30 seconds repeat pushing the eggs from the sides into the middle every 30 seconds till simply set, for a complete cooking time of about 5 minutes.

3.   Add the last word tablespoons raw egg and stir till eggs not look wet. Remove from warmness and season with salt and pepper as required. Serve immediately.

Nutrition

Calories 546 Carbs 5g Fat 40g Protein 39g Fiber 0g Net carbs 4g Sodium 586mg Cholesterol 1147mg

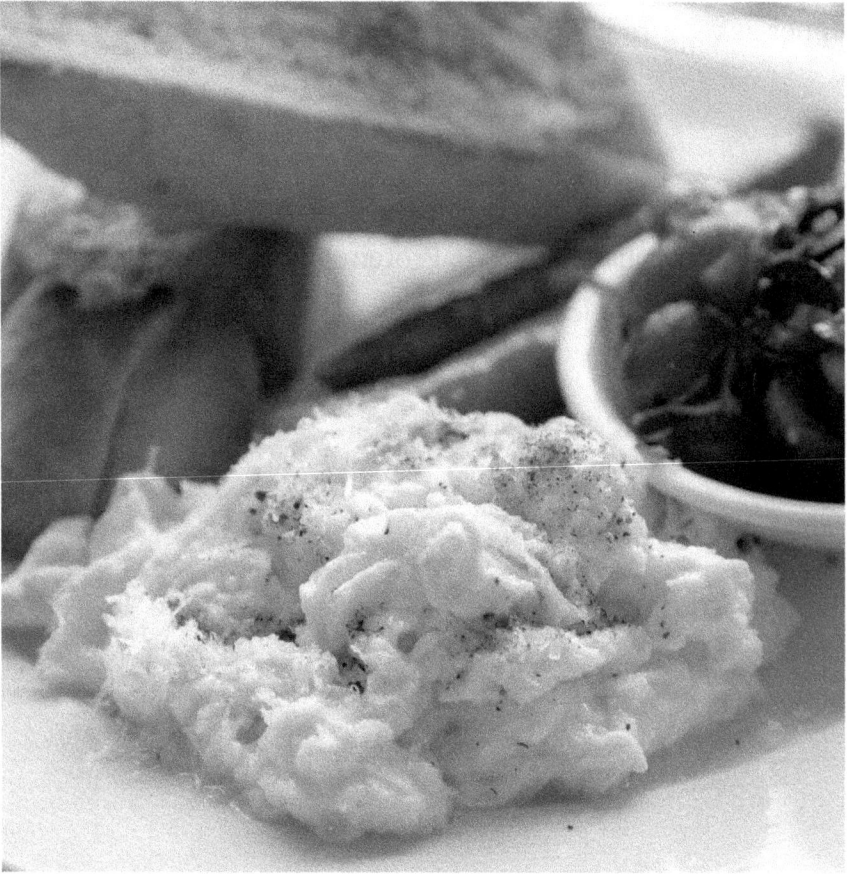

Baked Butternut-Squash Rigatoni

Ingredients

One large butternut squash

Three clove garlic

2 tbsp. olive oil

1 lb. rigatoni

1/2 c. heavy cream

3 c. shredded fontina

2 tbsp. chopped fresh sage

1 tbsp. salt

1 tsp. freshly ground pepper

1 c. panko breadcrumbs

Directions

1.   Set oven at 425 degrees. At an equivalent time, take an outsized bowl and toss garlic, squash, and vegetable oil for coating. Take a baking sheet and roast for about hour. Then calm for 20 minutes. Reduce oven to 350 degrees.

2.   Then, boil the salted water and cook rigatoni consistent with package directions. Drain and put aside .

3.   employing a blender, purée reserved squash with cream until smooth.

4.   Take an outsized bowl and blend squash puree with reserved rigatoni, 2 cups fontina, sage, salt, and pepper. Apply olive oil on the edges of the baking pan. Transfer rigatoni-squash mixture to plate.

5.   Take a little bowl, combine the remaining fontina and panko. Sprinkle over pasta and bake until golden brown,20 to 25 minutes.

Simple Caprese Sandwich

Ingredients

Sourdough bread, French or Vienna, Two slices, 192 grams
Mozzarella cheese

Whole milk 2 oz 56.7 grams

Tomatoes - Red, ripe, raw, year-round average

Four slices, medium (1/4" thick)

Instructions

Cut a large slice of sourdough in half (or use two small slices).
Top one slice with 1oz of sliced mozzarella and then two slices of
tomatoes. The flavor is mild, so season with salt pepper if
desired.

Nutrition

Calories707 Carbs104g Fat17g Protein34g Fiber5g Net

carbs99g Sodium1515mg Cholesterol45mg

Cottage Cheese Honey Toast

Ingredients

Whole-wheat bread-Commercially prepared-Two slice-56 grams

Cottage cheese- 1% milkfat-1 cup, (not packed)-226 grams

Honey-2 tbsp-42 grams

Directions

Toast bread to your liking. Spread with cottage cheese and drizzle with honey. Enjoy!

Nutrition

Calories432 Carbs65g Fat4g Protein35g Fiber3g Net carbs61g Sodium1174mg Cholesterol9mg

Pimento Cheese Sandwich

Ingredients

Pimento cheese-Pasteurized process-2 oz-56.7 grams Multi-grain bread-Four slices regular-104 grams

Directions

1.   Spread the pimento cheese on each side of bread. And then on the other slice of bread to form a sandwich. Enjoy!

Nutrition

Calories488 Carbs46g Fat22g Protein26g Fiber8g Net

carbs38g Sodium915mg Cholesterol53mg

Tomato Salad

Ingredients

Vinegar-Cider-2 2/3 tbsp-39.4 grams

Cucumber-Peeled, raw-Two medium-402 grams

Onions-Raw-1/2 large-75 grams

Tomatoes-Red, ripe, fresh, year-round average

Three medium whole (2-3/5" dia)-369 grams

Water-Plain, clean water-1/2 cup-118 grams

Directions

Peel and slice cucumbers into coins. Cut tomatoes into pieces. Dice red onion. Add vinegar and water and mix well.

Nutrition

Calories153 Carbs31g Fat1g Protein6g Fiber9g Net carbs22g Sodium32mg Cholesterol0mg

Tomato and Cheese Wrap

Ingredients

Tortillas-2 tortilla -92 grams

mayonnaise-like dressing-Regular, with salt-2 tbsp-29.4 grams

Tomatoes-Two medium whole -246 grams

Lettuce-2 cup shredded-144 grams

Cheddar cheese-2 oz-56.7 grams

Directions

1.   Lightly spread mayo on tortilla shell.

2.   Cut tomatoes however you like them.

3.   Layer ingredients, spreading them over the tortilla.

4.   Tuck up about an inch the side of the shell you've decided is the bottom and roll up the wrap. Enjoy!

Nutrition

Calories638 Carbs66g Fat32g Protein25g Fiber7g Net

carbs59g Sodium1236mg Cholesterol63mg

Peanut Butter Yogurt

Ingredients

Nonfat greek yogurt-1 cup-240 grams

Peanut butter-2 tbsp-32 grams

Vanilla extract-1 tsp-2.2 grams

Directions

Combine ingredients and enjoy it!

Nutrition

Calories345 Carbs16g Fat17g Protein32g Fiber2g Net

carbs15g Sodium223mg Cholesterol12mg

Peanut Butter & Carrots

Ingredients

Peanut butter-4 tbsp-64 grams

Carrots-2 cup chopped-256 grams

Directions

Spread peanut butter on carrots and enjoy!

Nutrition

Calories482 Carbs38g Fat33g Protein18g Fiber12g Net

carbs26g Sodium188mg Cholesterol0mg

Cucumber Tomato Salad with Tuna

Ingredients

Tomatoes-Two medium whole -246 grams

Lettuce-1 cup shredded-36 grams

Cucumber-With peel, raw-One cucumber-301 grams

Tuna-One can-165 grams

Directions

1.   Chop vegetables and lettuce.

2.   Toss together with the tuna and enjoy it!

Nutrition

Calories237 Carbs22g Fat2g Protein37g Fiber5g Net

carbs17g Sodium436mg Cholesterol59mg

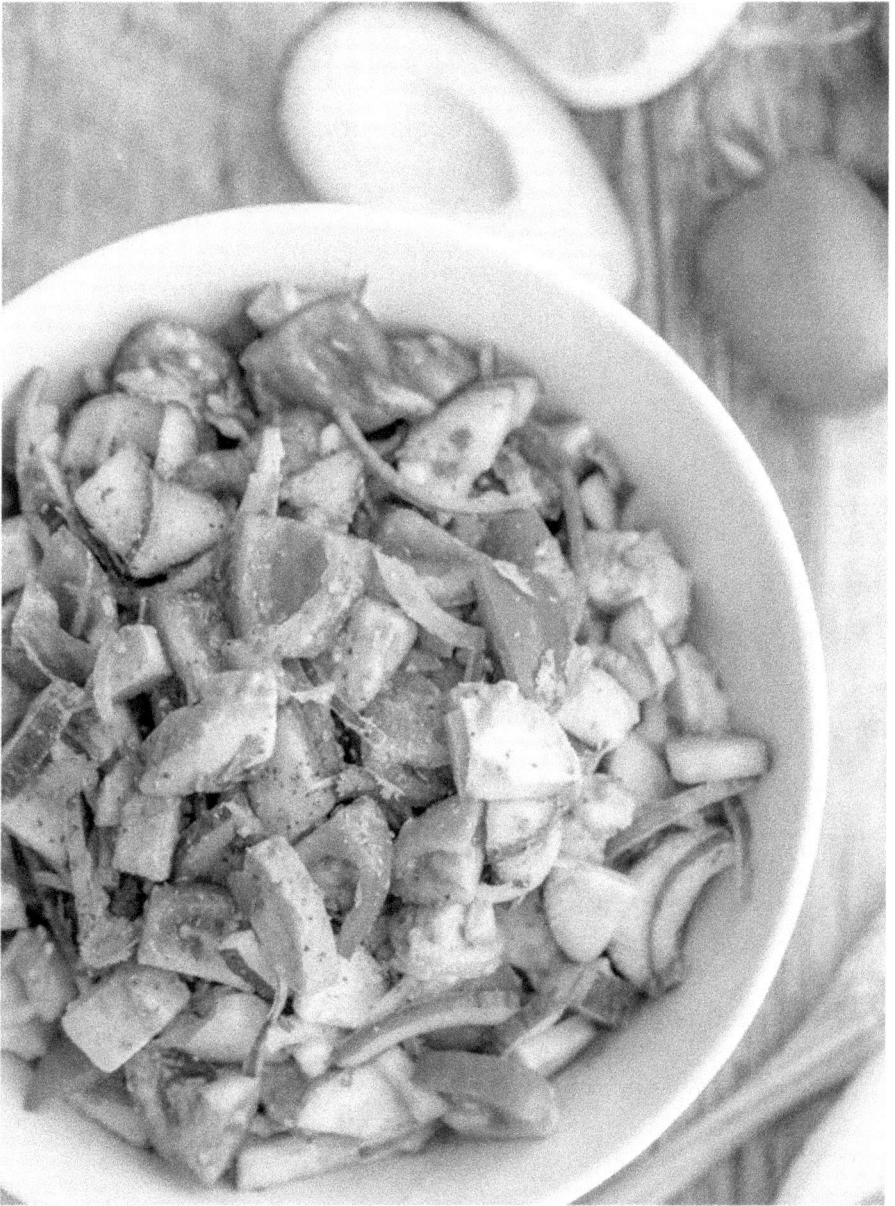

Peanut butter and Jelly

Ingredients

Multi-grain bread-Four slices regular-104 grams

Butter-Unsalted-2 tsp-9.5 grams

Peanut butter-Smooth style, without salt-3 tbsp-48 grams

Jams and preserves-2 tbsp-40 grams

Directions

1.   Toast the bread, and it's optionally. Drizzle1/2 teaspoon of butter on all sides of the bread.

2.   Spread butter on one side and jam on another side.

Nutrition

Calories742 Carbs83g Fat37g Protein25g Fiber11g Net

carbs73g Sodium418mg Cholesterol20mg

Chicken Scampi Pasta

Ingredients

1 pound of thinly-sliced chicken cutlets, cut into 1/2-inch-thick strips

Three tablespoons olive oil

Eight tablespoons unsalted butter, cubed Six cloves garlic, sliced

1/2 teaspoon crushed red pepper flakes

1/2 cup dry white wine

12 ounces angel hair pasta

One teaspoon lemon zest plus the juice of 1 large lemon 1/2 cup freshly grated Parmesan

1/2 cup chopped fresh Italian parsley

Directions

1.   Take a huge pot of salted water to a boil for the pasta. Sprinkle the chook with a couple of salts. Heat a huge skillet over medium-high warmth until hot, then upload the oil. Working in 2 batches, brown the chook until golden however not cooked through, 2 to a couple of minutes keep with batch. Remove the chicken to a plate.

2.   Melt four tablespoons of the butter within the skillet. Add the garlic and crimson pepper flakes and cook dinner until the garlic begins to show golden at the sides, 30 seconds to 1 minute. Add the wine, deliver to a simmer, and cook dinner till reduced by using half, approximately 2 minutes. Remove from the heat.

3.   Meanwhile, cook dinner the pasta till very hard, reserving 1 cup of the pasta water. Add the pasta and 3/four cup pasta water to the skillet alongside the hen, lemon peel and juice, and therefore the last four tablespoons butter. Return the skillet to medium-low warmness and gently stir the pasta until the butter is melted, including the last word 1/four pasta water if the pasta appears too dry. Remove the skillet from the heat, sprinkle with the cheese and parsley and toss before serving.

Apple-Cherry Pork Medallions

Ingredients

One pork tenderloin (1 pound)

One teaspoon minced fresh rosemary or 1/4 teaspoon dried rosemary, crushed

One teaspoon minced fresh thyme or 1/4 teaspoon dried thyme

1/2 teaspoon celery salt

One tablespoon olive oil

One large apple, sliced

2/3 cup unsweetened apple juice

Three tablespoons dried tart cherries

One tablespoon honey

One tablespoon cider vinegar

One package (8.8 ounces) ready-to-serve brown rice

Instructions

1. Cut tenderloin crosswise into 12 slices; sprinkle with rosemary, thyme and flavorer. during a huge skillet, heat oil over

medium-excessive heat. Brown pork on both sides; do away with from pan.

2.   In the equal skillet, combine apple, fruit juice, cherries, honey and vinegar. Boil it and stirring to loosen browned bits from pan. Reduce warmness; simmer, uncovered, 3-four minutes or simply till apple is tender.

3.   Return meat to the pan, turning to coat with sauce; cook, covered, 3-4 minutes or till meat is tender. Meanwhile, put together rice keep with package deal directions; serve with meat mixture.

Nutrition Facts

349 calories, 9g fat (2g saturated fat), 64mg cholesterol, 179mg sodium, 37g carbohydrate (16g sugars, 4g fibre), and 25g protein.

Butternut Turkey Soup

Ingredients

Three shallots, thinly sliced

One tsp of olive oil

3 cups of reduced-sodium chicken broth

3 cups of cubed peeled butternut squash (3/4-inch cubes) Two medium-sized red potatoes, cut into 1/2-inch cubes 1-1/2 cups of water

Two teaspoons of minced fresh thyme

1/2 teaspoon pepper

Two whole cloves

3 cups cubed cooked turkey breast

Instructions

1.   In a large-size saucepan coated with cooking spray, cook dinner shallots in oil over medium heat till tender. Stir within the broth, squash, potatoes, water, thyme and pepper.

2.   Place spices on a double thickness of cheesecloth; carry up corners of the material and tie with string to shape a bag. Stir into soup. bring back a boil. Reduce warmness; cowl and

simmer for 10-15 mins or till vegetables are tender. Stir in turkey; warmth through. Discard spice bag.

Nutrition

192 calories, 2g fat (0 saturated fat), 60mg cholesterol, 332mg sodium, 20g carbohydrate (3g sugars, 3g fibre), 25g protein.

Black Bean & Sweet Potato Rice Bowls

Ingredients

3/4 cup uncooked long-grain rice

1/4 teaspoon garlic salt

1-1/2 cups water

Three tablespoons olive oil, divided

One large sweet potato, peeled and diced

One medium red onion, finely chopped

4 cups chopped fresh kale (sturdy stems removed) One can (15 ounces) black beans, rinsed and drained Two tablespoons sweet chilli sauce Lime wedges, optional

Additional sweet chilli sauce, optional

Instructions

1.   Place rice, flavorer and water during a large saucepan; bring back a boil. Reduce heat; simmer, covered until liquid is absorbed and rice is tender 15-20 minutes. Remove from heat; let stand 5 minutes.

2.   At an equivalent time take an outsized pan and warmth two tablespoons oil over medium-high heat; saute sweet potato

8 minutes. Add onion; cook and stir until potato is tender 4-6 minutes. Add kale; cook and stir until tender, 3-5 minutes. Stir in beans; heat through.

3. Gently stir two tablespoons chilli sauce and remaining oil into rice; increase potato mixture. If you would like , serve with lime wedges and extra chilli sauce.

Nutrition

435 calories, 11g fat (2g saturated fat), 0 cholesterol, 405mg sodium, 74g carbohydrate (15g sugars, 8g fibre), 10g protein.

Pepper Ricotta Primavera

Ingredients

1 cup part-skim ricotta cheese

1/2 cup fat-free milk

Four teaspoons olive oil

One garlic clove, minced

1/2 teaspoon crushed red pepper flakes One medium green pepper, julienned One medium sweet red pepper, julienned One medium fresh yellow pepper, julienned One medium zucchini, sliced 1 cup frozen peas, thawed

1/4 teaspoon dried oregano

1/4 teaspoon dried basil

6 ounces fettuccine, cooked and drained

Instructions

1.   Whisk together ricotta cheese and milk; put aside. Take an outsized skillet, heat oil over medium heat. Add garlic and pepper; sauté 1 minute. Add subsequent seven ingredients. Cook and blend over medium heat until vegetables are crisp tender, about 5 minutes.

2.   Add cheese mixture to fettuccine; top with vegetables. Toss to coat. Serve immediately.

Nutrition

229 calories, 7g fat (3g saturated fat), 13mg cholesterol, 88mg sodium, 31g carbohydrate (6g sugars, 4g fibre), 11g protein.

Bow Ties with Sausage & Asparagus

Ingredients

3 cups of uncooked whole wheat bow tie pasta (about 8 ounces)

1 pound of asparagus, cut into 1-1/2-inch pieces

One package (19-1/2 ounces) Italian turkey sausage links, casings removed

One medium onion, chopped

Three garlic cloves, minced

1/4 cup shredded Parmesan cheese

Additional shredded Parmesan cheese, optional

Instructions

1.   In a 6-qt. Stockpot, prepare dinner pasta in line with package directions, including asparagus over the last 2-three minutes of cooking. Drain, reserving half cup pasta water; return pasta and asparagus to the pot.

2.   Meanwhile, during a big skillet, cook sausage, onion and garlic over medium heat until no pink, 6-8 minutes, breaking sausage into large crumbles. increase stockpot. Stir in 1/four cup

cheese and reserved pasta water as desired. Serve with additional cheese if desired.

Nutrition

247 calories, 7g fat (2g saturated fat), 36mg cholesterol, 441mg sodium, 28g carbohydrate (2g sugars, 4g fibre), 17g protein

Pork and Balsamic Strawberry Salad

Ingredients

One pork tenderloin (1 pound)

1/2 cup Italian salad dressing

1-1/2 cups halved fresh strawberries

Two tablespoons balsamic vinegar

Two teaspoons sugar

1/4 teaspoon salt

1/4 teaspoon pepper

Two tablespoons olive oil

1/4 cup chicken broth

One package about 5 ounces spring mix salad greens 1/2 cup crumbled goat cheese

Instructions

1.   Place pork during a shallow dish. Add salad dressing; flip for coating. Refrigerate and canopy for a minimum of eight hours. Mix strawberries, vinegar and sugar; cover and refrigerate.

2.   Preheat oven to 425°. Drain and wipe off meat , discarding marinade. Sprinkle with salt and pepper. during a large cast-iron or every other ovenproof skillet, warmness oil over medium-high warmness. Add beef; brown on all sides.

3.   Bake until a thermometer reads 145°, 15-20 minutes. Remove from skillet; permit or stand 5 min. Then, add broth to skillet; cook over medium warmth, stirring to loosen browned bits from pan. bring back a boil. Reduce warmth; add strawberry. Then heat it.

4.   Place green vegetables on a serving platter; sprinkle with cheese. Slice pork; found out over veggies. Top with strawberry mixture.

Nutrition

291 calories, 16g fat (5g saturated fat), 81mg cholesterol, 444mg sodium, 12g carbohydrate (7g sugars, 3g fibre), 26g protein.

Peppered Tuna Kabobs

Ingredients

1/2 cup frozen corn, thawed Four green onions, chopped One jalapeno pepper, seeded and chopped

Two tablespoons coarsely chopped fresh parsley Two tablespoons lime juice

1 pound tuna steaks, cut into 1-inch cubes One teaspoon coarsely ground pepper

Two large sweet red peppers, cut into 2x1-inch pieces

Instructions

1.   One medium mango, peeled and cut into 1-inch cubes

2.   For salsa, during a small bowl, combine the primary five ingredients; put aside.

3.   Rub tuna with pepper. On 4metal or soaked wooden skewers, alternately thread red peppers, tuna and mango.

4.   Place skewers on greased grill rack. Cook, covered, over medium heat, occasionally turning, until tuna is slightly pink in centre (medium-rare) and peppers are tender 10-12 minutes. Serve with salsa.

Nutrition

205 calories, 2g fat (0 saturated fat), 51mg cholesterol, 50mg sodium, 20g carbohydrate (12g sugars, 4g fibre), 29g protein.

Weeknight Chicken Chop Suey

Ingredients

Four teaspoons of olive oil

1 pound of boneless chicken breast side, cut into 1-inch cubes

1/2 teaspoon dried tarragon

1/2 teaspoon dried basil

1/2 teaspoon dried marjoram

1/2 teaspoon grated lemon zest

1-1/2 cups chopped carrots

1 cup unsweetened pineapple tidbits, drained (reserve juice)

One can (8 ounces) sliced water chestnuts, drained

One medium tart apple, chopped

1/2 cup chopped onion

1 cup cold water, divided

Three tablespoons unsweetened pineapple juice

Three tablespoons reduced-sodium teriyaki sauce

Two tablespoons cornstarch

3 cups hot cooked brown rice

Instructions

1.   In a massive cast-iron or another heavy skillet, heat oil at medium temperature. Add chicken, herbs and lemon zest; leave it until lightly browned. Add subsequent five ingredients. Stir in 3/four cup water, fruit juice and teriyaki sauce; bring back a boil. Reduce warmness; simmer covered till chicken is not any longer purple, and therefore the carrots are gentle 10-15 minutes.

2.   Combine cornstarch and remaining water. Gradually stir into hen mixture. Leave for boiling; cook and stir till thickened, about 2 minutes. Serve with rice.

Nutrition

330 calories, 6g fat, 42mg cholesterol, 227mg sodium, 50g carbohydrate (14g sugars, 5g fibre), 20g protein

Thai Chicken Pasta Skillet

Ingredients

6 ounces uncooked whole-wheat spaghetti Two teaspoons canola oil

One package (10 ounces) fresh sugar snap peas, trimmed and cut diagonally into thin strips

2 cups julienned carrots (about 8 ounces)

2 cups shredded cooked chicken

1 cup Thai peanut sauce

One medium cucumber, halved lengthwise, seeded and sliced diagonally

Chopped fresh cilantro, optional

Instructions

1.   Cook spaghetti according to package directions; drain.

2.   Then, during a large skillet, heat oil a medium-high heat. Add snap peas and carrots; stir-fry 6-8 minutes or until crisp tender. Add chicken, peanut sauce and spaghetti; heat through, tossing to mix.

3.   Transfer to a serving plate. Top with cucumber and, if desired, cilantro.

Nutrition Facts

403 calories, 15g fat (3g saturated fat), 42mg cholesterol, 432mg sodium, 43g carbohydrate (15g sugars, 6g fibre), 25g protein

Spinach-Orzo Salad with Chickpeas

Ingredients

One 14-1/2 ounces reduced-sodium chicken broth 1-1/2 cups of uncooked whole wheat orzo pasta 4 cups of fresh baby spinach

2 cups of grape tomatoes, halved

Two cans (15 ounces each) of chickpeas or garbanzo beans, rinsed and drained

3/4 cup chopped fresh parsley

Two green onions, chopped

DRESSING:

1/4 cup olive oil

Three tablespoons lemon juice

3/4 teaspoon salt

1/4 teaspoon garlic powder

1/4 teaspoon hot pepper sauce

1/4 teaspoon pepper

Instructions

1.   Take an outsized saucepan and convey broth to a boil. Stir in orzo; return to a boil. Reduce heat; simmer, covered, until hard, 8-10 minutes.

2.   Take an outsized pan and add spinach and warm orzo, allowing the spinach to wilt slightly. Add tomatoes, chickpeas, parsley and green onions.

3.   Whisk together dressing ingredients. Toss with salad.

Nutrition

122 calories, 5g fat, 0 cholesterol, 259mg sodium, 16g carbohydrate (1g sugars, 4g fibre), 4g protein. Diabetic Exchanges: 1 starch, one fat.

Roasted Chicken Thighs with Peppers & Potatoes

Ingredients

2 pounds red potatoes (about six medium)

Two large sweet red peppers

Two large green peppers

Two medium onions

Two tablespoons olive oil, divided

Four teaspoons minced fresh thyme or 1-1/2 teaspoons dried thyme, divided

Three teaspoons minced fresh rosemary or one teaspoon dried rosemary, crushed, divided

Eight boneless skinless chicken thighs (about 2 pounds)

1/2 teaspoon salt

1/4 teaspoon pepper

Instructions

1.   Preheat oven to 450°. Cut potatoes, peppers and onions into 1-in. Pieces. Place vegetables during a roasting pan. Drizzle

with one tablespoon oil; sprinkle with two teaspoons each thyme and rosemary and toss to coat. Place chicken over greens. Brush chicken with remaining oil; sprinkle with remaining thyme and rosemary. Drizzle vegetables and chicken with salt and pepper.

2.   Roast until a thermometer inserted in chicken reads 170° and green vegetables are tender 35-40 minutes.

Nutrition Facts

308 calories, 12g fat (3g saturated fat), 76mg cholesterol, 221mg sodium, 25g carbohydrate (5g sugars, 4g fibre), 24g protein. Diabetic Exchanges: 3 lean meat, one starch, one vegetable, 1/2 fat.

Spiced Split Pea Soup

Ingredients

1 cup dried green split peas

Two medium potatoes, chopped

Two medium carrots, halved and thinly sliced

One medium onion, chopped

One celery rib, thinly sliced

Three garlic cloves, minced

Three bay leaves

Four teaspoons curry powder

One teaspoon ground cumin

1/2 teaspoon coarsely ground pepper

1/2 teaspoon ground coriander

One carton (32 ounces) reduced-sodium chicken broth One can (28 ounces) diced tomatoes, undrained

Instructions

1.   In a 4-qt. Slow cooker combines the primary 12 ingredients. Cook, covered, on low until peas are tender, 8-10 hours.

2.   Stir in tomatoes; heat through. Discard bay leaves.

Nutrition Facts

139 calories, 0 fat (0 saturated fat), 0 cholesterol, 347mg sodium, 27g carbohydrate (7g sugars, 8g fibre), 8g protein. Diabetic Exchanges: 1 starch, one lean meat, one vegetable.

Escarole and Bean Soup

Ingredients

Two tablespoons olive oil

Two chopped garlic cloves

1 pound of escarole, chopped

Salt

4 cups of low-salt broth chicken

1 can of cannellini bean

1 (1-ounce) piece of Parmesan

Freshly ground black pepper

Six teaspoons extra-virgin olive oil

Directions

1.   Heat vegetable oil during a big heavy pot at normal heat.
Add the garlic and sauté till fragrant, for 15 seconds. Add the
escarole and sauté till wilted, for 2 min. Add salt. Add the
chicken, beans, then Parmesan cheese. Cover and simmer till
the beans are heated through, approximately five minutes —
season with salt and pepper, to taste.

2.   Ladle the soup into six bowls. Sprinkle one teaspoon extra-virgin vegetable oil over each. Serve with crusty bread.

Creamy Shrimp Salad

Serving: 4

Prep Time: 20 minutes

Cook Time: 5 minutes

Ingredients:

4 pounds large shrimp

1 lemon, quartered

3 cups celery stalks, chopped

1 red onion, chopped

2 cups mayonnaise

2 tablespoons white wine vinegar

1 teaspoon Dijon mustard

Salt and pepper as needed

How To:

1.   Take a large pan and place it over medium heat.

2.   Add water (salted) and bring water to boil.

3. Add shrimp and lemon, cook for 3 minutes.

4. Let them cool.

5. Peel and de-vein the shrimps.

6. Take a large bowl and add cooked shrimp alongside remaining ingredients.

7. Stir well.

8. Serve immediately or chilled!

Nutrition (Per Serving)

Calories: 153

Fat: 5g

Carbohydrates: 8g

Protein: 19g

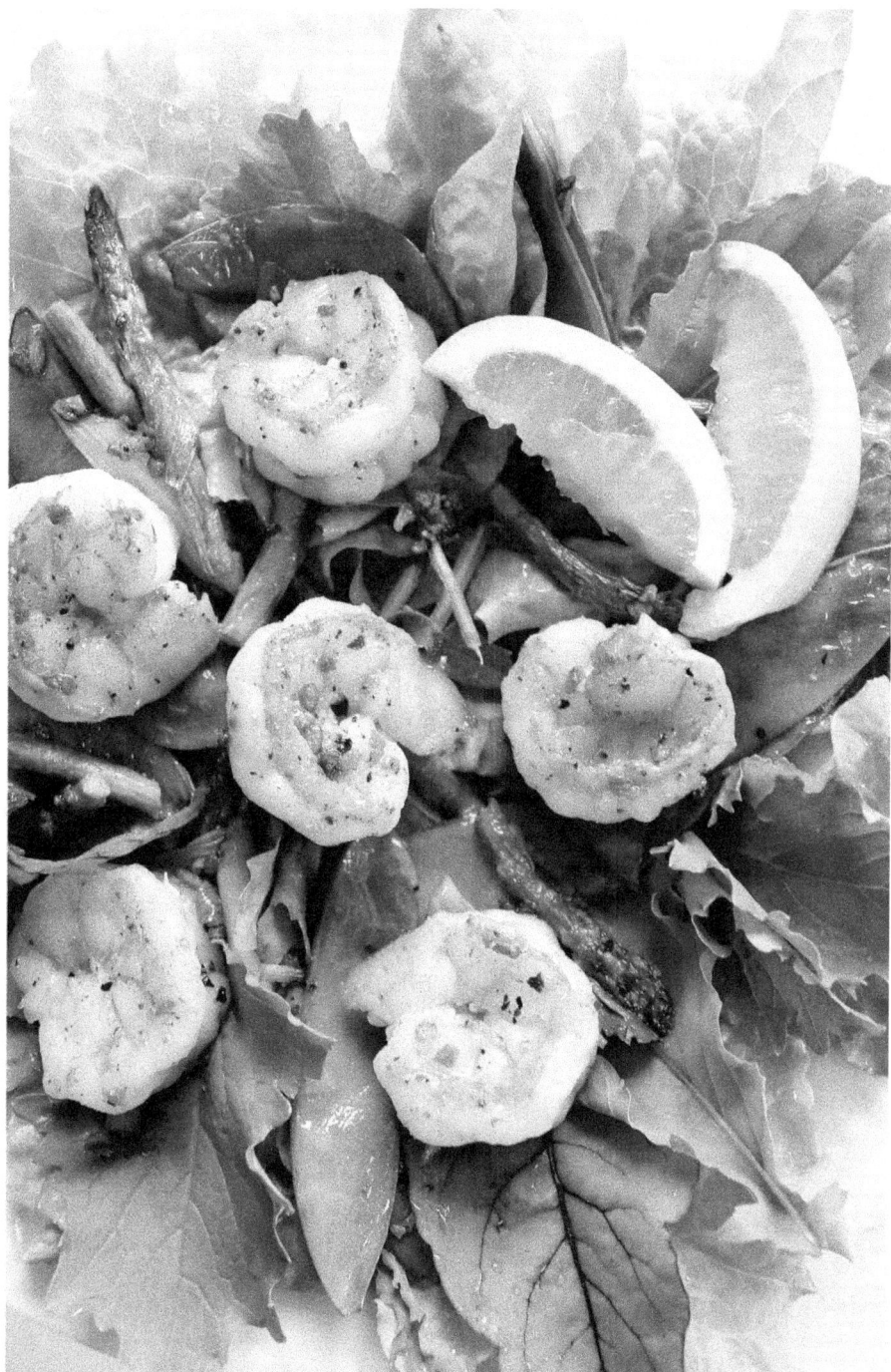

Passionate Quinoa and Black Bean Salad

Serving: 6

Prep Time: 5 minutes

Cook Time: 15 minutes

Ingredients:

1 cup uncooked quinoa

1 can 15 ounce black beans, drained and rinsed 1/3 cup cilantro, chopped

1 tablespoon olive oil

1 clove garlic, minced

Juice from 1 lime

Salt and pepper as needed

How To:

1.   Cook quinoa according to the package instructions.

2.   Transfer quinoa to a medium bowl and let it cool for 10 minutes.

3.   Add remaining ingredients and toss well.

4.   Serve and enjoy!

Nutrition (Per Serving)

Calories: 188

Fat: 4g

Carbohydrates: 29g

Protein: 8g

Zucchini Noodle Salad

Serving: 3

Prep Time: 15 minutes

Cook Time: nil

Ingredients:

2 large zucchini, spiralized/peeled into thin strips

1 small tomato, diced

¼ red onion, sliced thinly

1 large avocado, diced

½ cup olive oil

¼ cup balsamic vinegar

1 garlic clove, minced

2 teaspoons Dijon mustard

Salt and pepper to taste

¼ cup blue cheese, crumbles

How To:

1.   Take a large bowl and add zucchini noodles, onion, tomato, avocado.

2.   Take a small bowl and whisk in olive oil, vinegar, mustard, garlic, salt and pepper.

3.   Drizzle over salad and toss.

4.   Divide into serving bowls and top with blue cheese crumbles.

5.   Enjoy!

Nutrition (Per Serving)

Calories: 770

Fat: 74

Carbohydrates: 12g

Protein: 8g

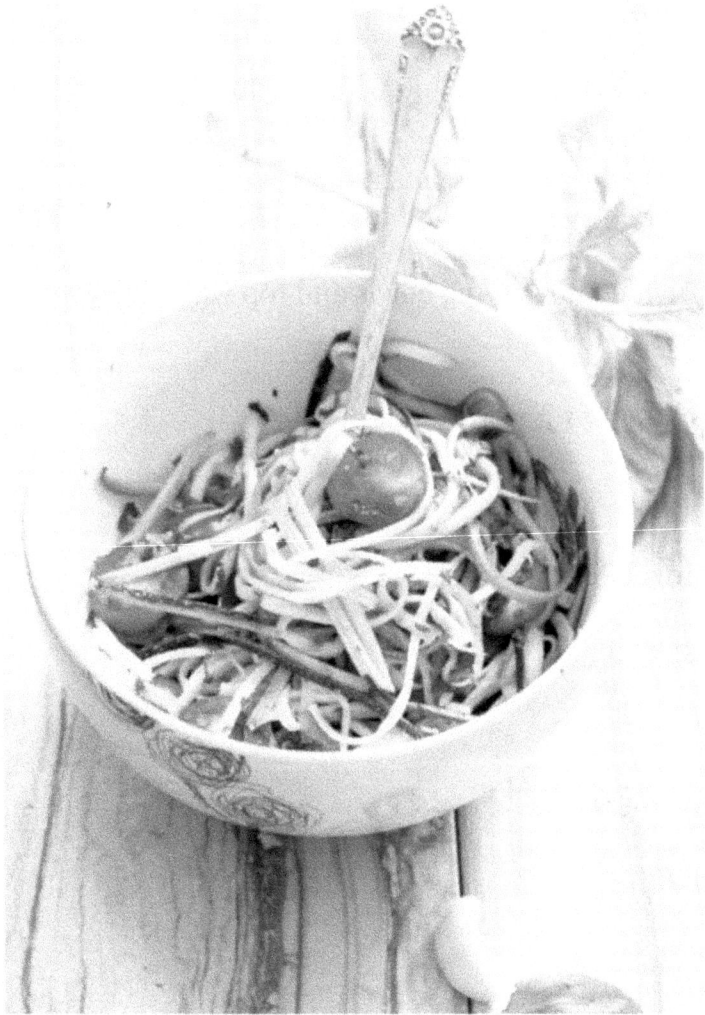

Onion and Orange Healthy Salad

Serving: 3

Prep Time: 10 minutes

Cook Time: nil

Ingredients:

6 large oranges

3 tablespoons red wine vinegar

6 tablespoons olive oil

1 teaspoon dried oregano

1 red onion, thinly sliced

1 cup olive oil

¼ cup fresh chives, chopped Ground black pepper

How To:

1.   Peel the oranges and cut each of them in 4-5 crosswise slices.

2.   Transfer the oranges to a shallow dish.

3.   Drizzle vinegar, olive oil and sprinkle oregano.

4.   Toss.

5.   Chill for 30 minutes.

6.   Arrange sliced onion and black olives on top.

7.   Decorate with additional sprinkle of chives and fresh grind of pepper.

8.   Serve and enjoy!

Nutrition (Per Serving)

Calories: 120

Fat: 6g

Carbohydrates: 20g

Protein: 2g

Stir Fried Almond and Spinach

Serving: 2

Prep Time: 10 minutes

Cook Time: 15 minutes

Ingredients:

34 pounds spinach

3 tablespoons almonds

Salt to taste

1 tablespoon coconut oil

How To:

1.   Add oil to a large pot and place on high heat.

2.   Add spinach and let it cook, stirring frequently.

3.   Once the spinach is cooked and tender, season with salt and stir.

4.   Add almonds and enjoy!

Nutrition (Per Serving)

Calories: 150

Fat: 12g

Carbohydrates: 10g

Protein: 8g

Cilantro and Avocado Platter

Serving: 6

Prep Time: 10 minutes

Cook Time: nil

Ingredients:

2 avocados, peeled, pitted and diced

1 sweet onion, chopped

1 green bell pepper, chopped

1 large ripe tomato, chopped

¼ cup fresh cilantro, chopped

½ lime, juiced

Salt and pepper as needed

How To:

1.   Take a medium sized owl and add onion, bell pepper, tomato, avocados, lime and cilantro.

2.   Mix well and give it a toss.

3. Season with salt and pepper according to your taste.

4. Serve and enjoy!

Nutrition (Per Serving)

Calories: 126

Fat: 10g

Carbohydrates: 10g

Protein: 2g

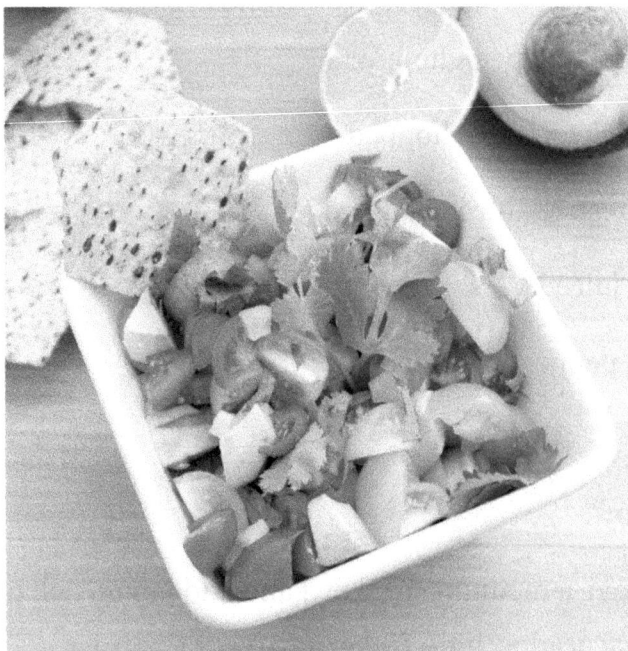

Chicken Breast Salad

Serving: 4

Prep Time: 25 minutes

Cook Time: 30-55 minutes

Ingredients:

3 ½ ounces chicken breast

2 tablespoons spinach

1 ¾ ounces lettuces

1 bell pepper

2 tablespoons olive oil

Lemon juice to taste

How To:

1.   Boil chicken breast without adding salt, cut the meat into small strips.

2.   Put the spinach in boiling water for a few minutes, cut into small strips.

3.   Cut pepper in strips as well.

4.   Add everything to a bowl and mix with juice and oil.

5.   Serve!

Nutrition (Per Serving)

Calories: 100

Fat: 11g

Carbohydrates: 3g

Protein: 6g

Broccoli Salad

Serving: 1

Prep Time: 5 minutes

Cook Time: 10 minutes

Ingredients:

broccoli florets

2 red onions, sliced

1-ounce bacon, chopped into small pieces

1 cup coconut cream

1 teaspoon sesame seeds Salt

How To:

1.   Cook bacon in hot oil until crispy.

2.   Cook onions in fat left from the bacon.

3.   Take a pan of boiling water and add broccoli florets, boil for a few minutes.

4.   Take a salad bowl and add bacon pieces, onions, broccoli florets, coconut cream and salt.

5. Toss well and top with sesame seeds.

6. Enjoy!

Nutrition (Per Serving)

Calories: 280

Fat: 26g

Carbohydrates: 8g

Protein: 10g

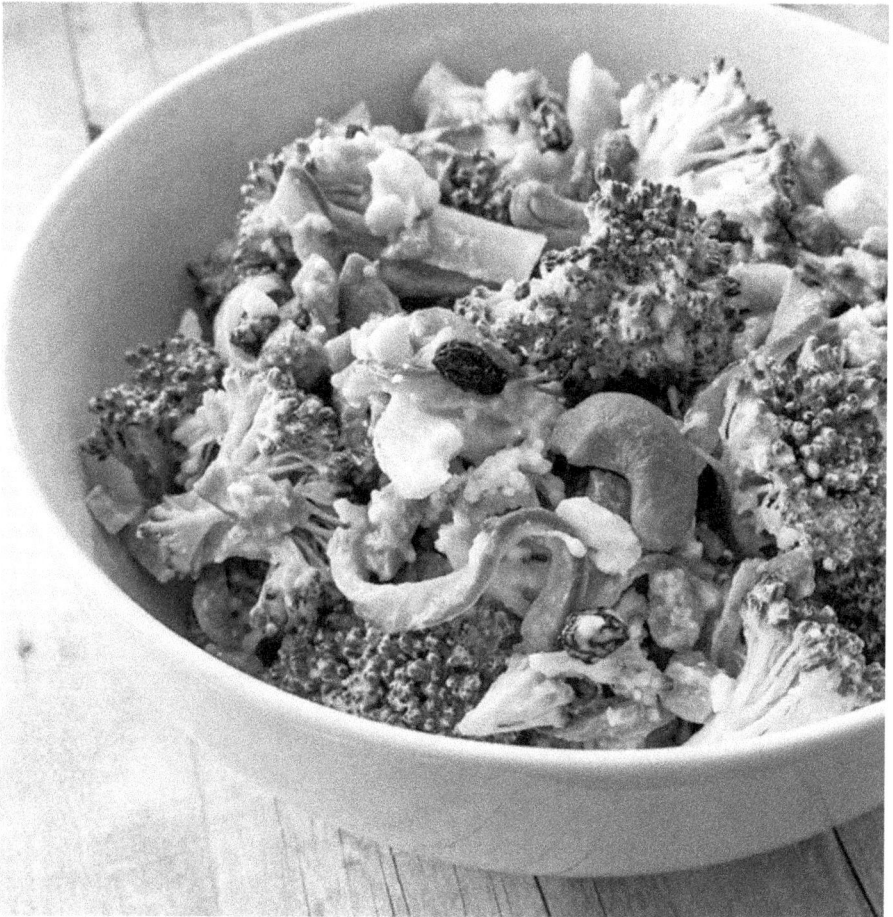

Hearty Quinoa and Fruit Salad

Serving: 5

Prep Time: 5 minutes

Cook Time: 10 minutes

Ingredients:

3 ½ ounces Quinoa

3 peaches, diced

1 ½ ounces toasted hazelnuts, chopped

Handful of mint, chopped

Handful of parsley, chopped

2 tablespoons olive oil

Zest of 1 lemon

Juice of 1 lemon

How To:

1.   Take medium sized saucepan and add quinoa.

2.   Add 1 ¼ cups of water and bring it to a boil over medium-high heat.

3.   Reduce the heat to low and simmer for 20 minutes.

4.   Drain any excess liquid.

5.   Add fruits, herbs, hazelnuts to the quinoa.

6.   Allow it to cool and season.

7.   Take a bowl and add olive oil, lemon zest and lemon juice.

8.   Pour the mixture over the salad and give it a mix.

9.   Enjoy!

Nutrition (Per Serving)

Calories: 148

Fat: 8g

Carbohydrates: 16g

Protein: 5g

Amazing Quinoa and Black Bean Salad

Serving: 4

Prep Time: 5 minutes

Cook Time: 2-3 minutes

Ingredients:

1 cup uncooked quinoa

1 can 15-ounce black beans, drained and rinsed 1/3 cup cilantro, chopped

1 tablespoon olive oil

1 clove garlic, minced

Juice from 1 lime

Salt and pepper as needed

How To:

1.   Cook quinoa according to package instructions.

2.   Transfer quinoa to a medium bowl and allow it to cool for 10 minutes.

3.   Add the rest of the ingredients and toss.

4.   Serve and enjoy!

5.   Enjoy!

Nutrition (Per Serving)

Calories: 188

Fat: 4g

Carbohydrates: 29g

Protein: 8g

Authentic Mediterranean Pearl and Couscous

Serving: 4

Prep Time: 15 minutes

Cook Time: 10 minutes

Ingredients:

For the Vinaigrette

1 large lemon, juiced

1/3 cup extra virgin olive oil

1 teaspoon dill weed

1 teaspoon garlic powder

Salt and pepper as needed

For Israeli Couscous

2 cups Pearl Couscous

Extra virgin olive oil

2 cups grape tomatoes, halved

Water as needed

1/3 cup red onions, chopped

½ English Cucumber, chopped

15 ounces chickpeas

14 ounce (can) fresh artichoke hearts, chopped ½ cup kalamata olives, pitted

15-20 pieces fresh basil leaves, torn and chopped

3 ounces fresh baby mozzarella cheese

How To:

1.   Start by preparing the vinaigrette. Take a bowl and add the ingredients listed under vinaigrette.

2.   Mix them well and keep it on the side.

3.   Take a medium sized heavy pot and place it over medium heat.

4.   Add 2 tablespoons of olive oil and allow it to heat up.

5.   Add couscous and keep cooking until golden brown.

6.   Add 3 cups of boiling water and cook the couscous according to package instructions.

7.   Once done, drain in a colander and keep on the side.

8.   Take another large sized mixing bowl and add the rest of the ingredients, except cheese and basil.

9.   Add the cooked couscous and basil to the mix and mix everything well.

10.   Give the vinaigrette a nice stir and whisk it into the couscous salad.

11.   Mix well.

12.   Adjust the seasoning as required.

13.   Add mozzarella cheese.

14.   Garnish with some basil.

15.   Enjoy!

Nutrition (Per Serving)

Calories: 393

Fat: 13g

Carbohydrates: 57g

Protein: 13g

Mesmerizing Fruit Bowl

Serving: 1

Prep Time: 30 minutes

Cook Time: nil

Ingredients:

2 fresh ripe mangoes

2 cups pineapple chunks

Fresh pineapple tips

1 banana, sliced

1-2 cups fresh papaya, cubed

1 kiwi fruit, cubed

2 cups seedless grapes, halved

¼ cup coconut milk

2 tablespoons lime juice

3-4 tablespoons sugar

Strawberries, cranberries or raspberries as topping

How To:

1.   Slice the fruits above, except the contrasting red ones such as dried cranberries, raspberries and strawberries.

2.   Add them to your mixing bowl and drizzle a bit of lime juice on top.

3.   Stir well and sprinkle a bit of sugar on top, give it a nice stir.

4.   Allow it to chill for 30 minutes and serve the salad with a bit of coconut milk.

5.   Season the sweetness accordingly and top it with some cranberries, raspberries and strawberries.

6.   Enjoy!

Nutrition (Per Serving)

Calories: 209

Fat: 0g

Carbohydrates: 43g

Protein: 2g

Tangy Strawberry Salad

Serving: 4

Prep Time: 15 minutes

Cook Time: nil

Ingredients:

4 slices bacon, cooked and crumbled

10 large strawberries, stem removed and sliced

4 cups baby spinach

1 avocado, chopped

For Dressing

Zest of 1 lemon

¼ red onion, minced

¼ cup red wine vinegar

1 tablespoon Dijon mustard

1 lemon, juiced

1 teaspoon poppy seed

½ cup extra light olive oil

How To:

1.   Add all the dressing ingredients to a blender and blend until you have a smooth mixture (except poppy seeds).

2.   Stir in poppy seeds after blending.

3.   Take a large bowl and toss strawberries, bacon, spinach and avocado.

4.   Mix well and drizzle the dressing on top.

5.   Serve and enjoy!

Nutrition (Per Serving)

Calories: 96

Fat: 1g

Carbohydrates: 22g

Protein: 3g

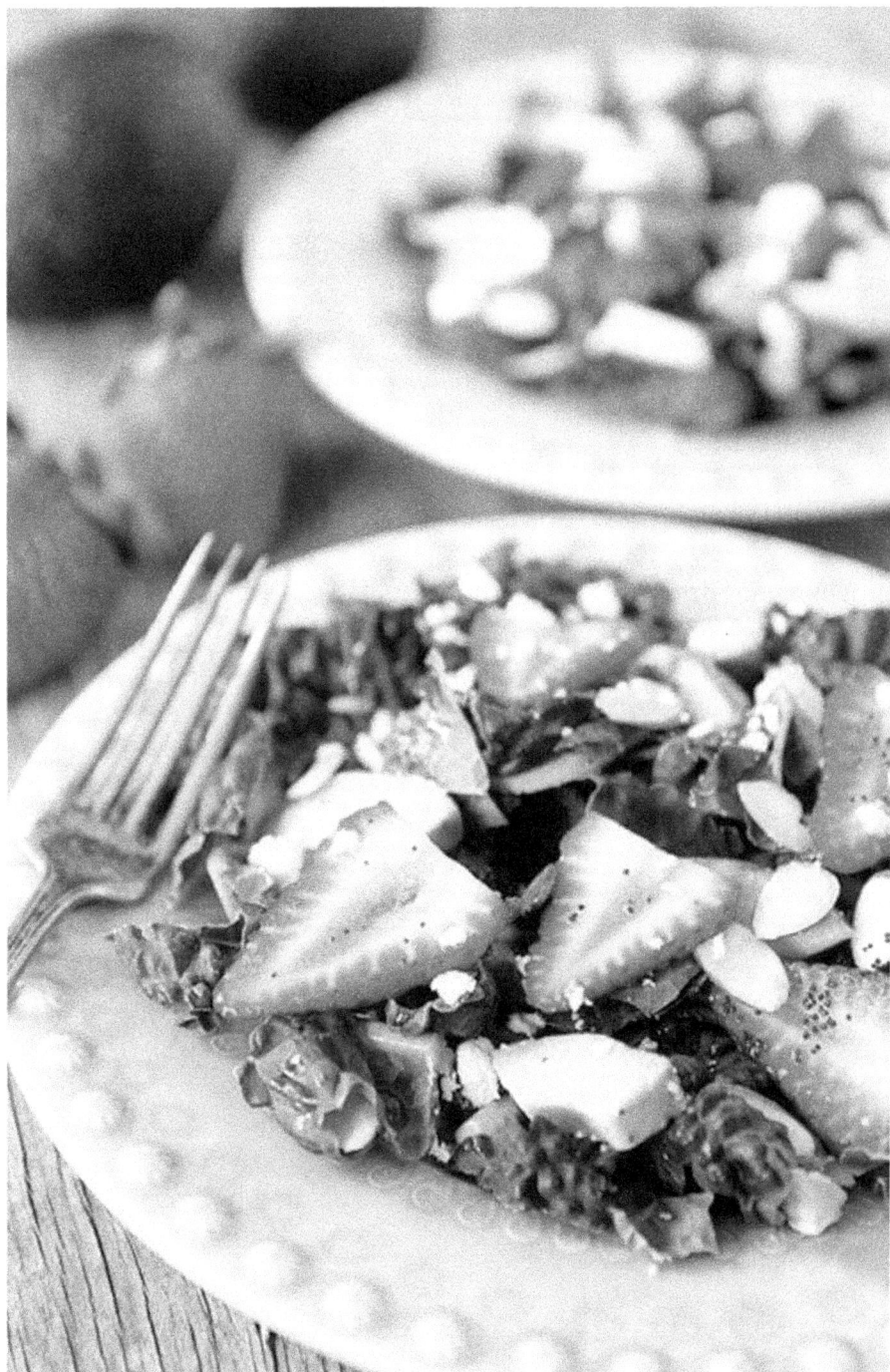

Peachful Applesauce Salad

Serving: 6

Prep Time: 15 minutes

Cook Time: nil

Ingredients:

1 cup diet lemon lime-soda

1 pack sugar-free fruit mixed peach gelatin

1 cup unsweetened applesauce

2 cups coconut whip cream

1/8 teaspoon ground nutmeg

1/8 teaspoon vanilla extract

1 fresh peach, peeled and chopped

How To:

1.   Take a saucepan and bring the soda to a boil over medium heat.

2.   Remove heat.

3. Stir in sugar-free peach gelatin until dissolved.

4. Add applesauce and stir.

5. Let it chill until partially set.

6. Fold in whipped topping and vanilla extract.

7. Fold in the peach and wait until firm.

8. Serve and enjoy!

Nutrition (Per Serving)

Calories: 354

Fat: 17g

Carbohydrates: 37g

Protein: 15g

The Citrus Lover's Salad

Serving: 16

Prep Time: 10 minutes

Cook Time: nil

Ingredients:

1 medium zucchini, julienned

½ cup olive oil

1 medium red onion, sliced

1 cup fresh broccoli, cut into florets

1 cup fresh cauliflower florets

1/8 teaspoon pepper

1 medium cucumber, halved and sliced ¼ cup white wine vinegar

1 teaspoon dried oregano

1 medium carrot, julienned

½ teaspoon ground mustard

¼ teaspoon garlic powder

1/8 teaspoon celery salt

How To:

1. Add olives and veggies to a small bowl.

2. Take another bowl and whisk in vinegar, seasoning, oil.

3. Pour the mixture over veggies and toss.

4. Let sit for 3 hours.

5. Serve and enjoy!

Nutrition (Per Serving)

Calories: 72

Fat: 7g

Carbohydrates: 2g

Protein: 2g

Wicked Vanilla Fruit Salad

Serving: 5

Prep Time: 10 minutes

Cook Time: nil

Ingredients:

8 cans mandarin orange, drained

4 packs instant vanilla pudding mix

6 cans pineapple chunks

10 medium red apples, chopped

How To:

1.   Drain pineapples, making sure to reserve the liquid.

2.   Keep them on the side.

3.   Add cold water to the juice to make 6 cups liquid in total.

4.   Whisk the juice mix and pudding mix into a large bowl for about 2 minutes.

5. Let it stand for 2 minutes until soft-set.

6. Stir in apples, oranges and reserved pineapple.

7. Chill in fridge and serve.

8. Enjoy!

Nutrition (Per Serving)

Calories: 33

Fat: 0g

Carbohydrates: 8g

Protein: 0g

Green Papaya Salad

Serving: 6

Prep Time: 10 minutes

Cook Time: nil

Ingredients:

10 small shrimps, dried

2 small red Thai Chilies

1 garlic clove, peeled

¼ cup tamarind juice

1 tablespoon palm sugar

1 tablespoon Thai fish sauce, low sodium

1 lime, cut into 1-inch pieces

4 cherry tomatoes, halved

3 long beans, trimmed into 1-inch pieces

1 carrot, coarsely shredded

½ English cucumber, coarsely chopped and seeded 1/6 small green cabbage, cored and thinly sliced

1-pound unripe green papaya, quartered, seeded and shredded using a mandolin

3 tablespoons unsalted roasted peanuts

How To:

1.   Take a mortar and pestle and crush your shrimp alongside garlic, chilies.

2.   Add tamarind juice, fish sauce and palm sugar.

3.   Squeeze the juice from the lime pieces and pour 3 quarts over the mortar.

4.   Grind the mixture in the mortar to make a dressing, keep the dressing on the side.

5.   Take a bowl, add the remaining ingredients (excluding the peanut), making sure to add the papaya last.

6.   Use a spoon and stir in the dressing.

7.   Mix the vegetables and fruit and coat them well.

8.   Transfer to your serving dish.

9.   Garnish with some peanuts and lime pieces.

10.   Enjoy!

Nutrition (Per Serving)

Calories: 316

Fat: 13g

Carbohydrates: 5g

Protein: 11g

Pineapple, Papaya and Mango Delight

Serving: 2

Prep Time: 20 minutes

Cook Time: nil

Ingredients:

1-pound fresh pineapple, peeled and cut into chunks mango, peeled, pitted and cubed papayas, peeled, seeded and cubed

tablespoons fresh lime juice

¼ cup fresh mint leaves, chopped

How To:

1. Take a large bowl and add the listed ingredients.

2.   Toss well to coat.

3.   Put in fridge and chill. Serve and enjoy!

Nutrition (Per Serving)

Calories: 292

Fat: 11g

Carbohydrates: 42g

Protein: 8g

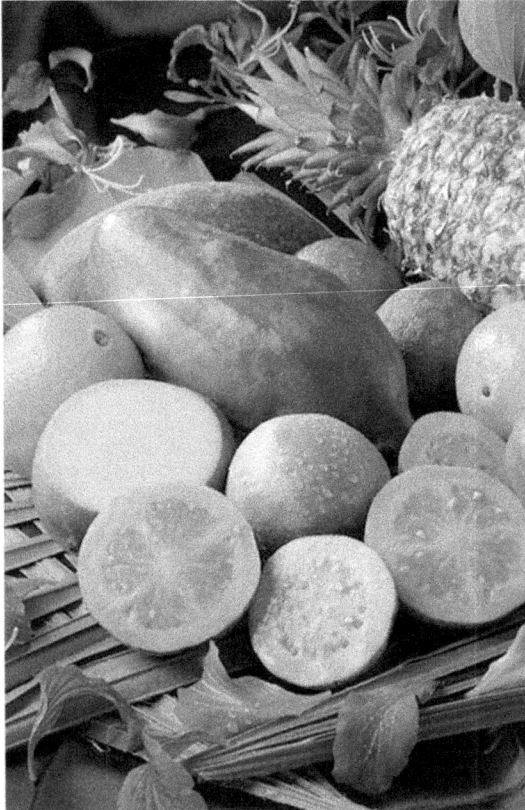

Cashew and Green Apple Salad

Serving: 2

Prep Time: 15 minutes

Cook Time: nil

Ingredients:

½ large apple, cored and sliced

2 cups mixed fresh greens

1 tablespoon unsalted cashews

1 tablespoon apple cider vinegar

How To:

1.   Take a serving bowl and add apple, cashews and greens.

2.   Drizzle apple cider vinegar on top.

3.   Serve immediately!

Nutrition (Per Serving)

Calories: 118

Fat: 4g

Carbohydrates: 19g

Protein: 3g

Watermelon and Tomato Mix

Serving: 2

Prep Time: 20 minutes

Cook Time: nil

Ingredients:

1 large red tomato, cubed

1 large yellow tomato, cubed

2 cups fresh watermelon, peeled, seeded and cubed

Dressing

¼ cup olive oil

¼ cup rice wine vinegar

2 teaspoons honey

2 tablespoons chili garlic sauce

1 tablespoon fresh lemon basil, chopped Salt and pepper as needed

How To:

1.   Take a large bowl and add all the salad ingredients.

2.   Take another bowl and add the dressing ingredients.

3.   Beat well until combined.

4.   Pour dressing over salad and toss.

5.   Serve and enjoy!

Nutrition (Per Serving)

Calories: 87

Fat: 7g

Carbohydrates: 7g

Protein: 0.6g

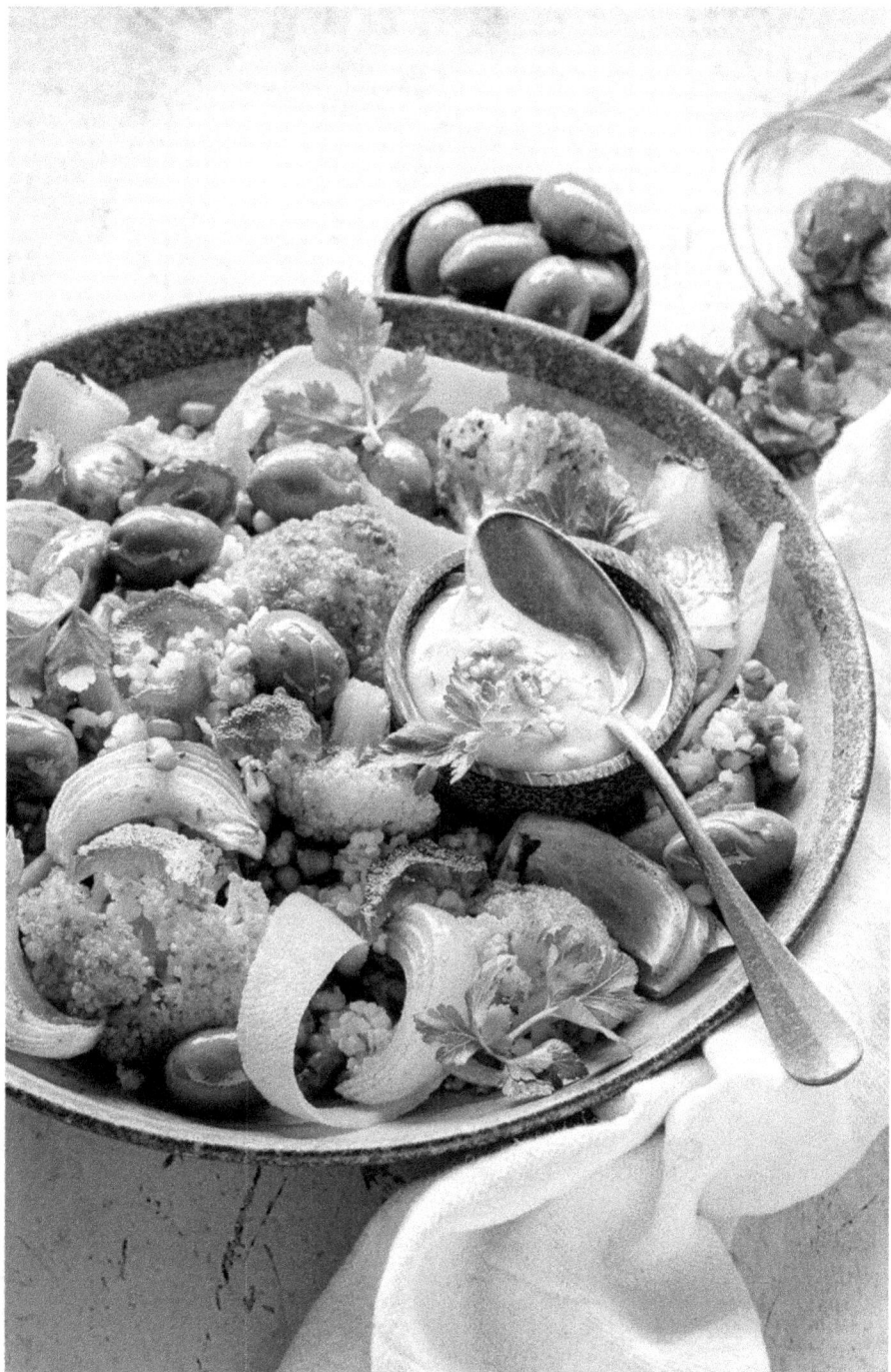

www.ingramcontent.com/pod-product-compliance
Lightning Source LLC
Chambersburg PA
CBHW070723030426
42336CB00013B/1906